Table of Contents

1 **The Origins of Fenbendazol**
2 **How Fenbendazole and Ivermectin Work Against Cancer**
3 **Reviewing the Scientific Studies and Evidence**
4 **Setting Up a Fenbendazole or Ivermectin Protocol**
5 **Integrating the Protocol with Conventional and Alternative Therapies**
6 **The Future of Repurposed Drugs in Cancer Treatment**

Chapter 1: The Origins of Fenbendazole and Ivermectin

A Surprising Connection to Cancer Treatment

Fenbendazole and ivermectin were never designed with cancer treatment in mind. Their origins lie in the realm of parasitic disease control, where they have been used extensively to combat infections in both animals and humans. Despite their intended purposes, researchers and patients alike have begun to explore their potential in a completely different context—fighting cancer.

Fenbendazole belongs to a class of drugs known as benzimidazoles, primarily used in veterinary medicine to treat parasitic infections in livestock, pets, and even zoo animals. It works by disrupting the metabolism of parasites, effectively starving them and leading to their elimination. Meanwhile, ivermectin, a groundbreaking discovery that won a Nobel Prize, has been used in human medicine to treat conditions like river blindness and scabies, as well as in veterinary medicine for a broad range of parasites.

A Growing Curiosity

In recent years, anecdotal reports and small-scale research have sparked curiosity about whether these drugs could be repurposed for cancer treatment. Patients looking for alternative approaches have shared stories of unexpected tumor shrinkage after incorporating one or both of these medications into their regimen. Scientists, intrigued by these reports, have started investigating how these drugs interact with cancer cells at a molecular level.

The idea of repurposing existing drugs for new uses is not new—many widely accepted treatments today were originally intended for completely different conditions. The emerging interest in fenbendazole and ivermectin as potential cancer-fighting agents fits into this broader trend, where overlooked compounds are given fresh scrutiny under the lens of modern oncology.

A Drug for Animals, a Potential Breakthrough for Humans

The story of fenbendazole begins in the world of veterinary medicine. Developed as part of a class of drugs called benzimidazoles, it was designed to target and eliminate parasites in animals. For decades, it has been a go-to treatment for livestock, household pets, and even zoo animals, effectively ridding them of intestinal worms and other parasites that threaten their health. Unlike many medications that require extensive monitoring, fenbendazole is widely regarded as safe, with minimal side effects, making it an essential tool for veterinarians.

Despite its effectiveness in animal health, fenbendazole remained largely unknown outside of veterinary circles. It wasn't until recent years that some patients with cancer began experimenting with it, believing it might have unintended benefits beyond its original purpose. This shift in attention was sparked by scattered reports of individuals who, after taking fenbendazole for parasitic infections, noticed unexpected improvements in their cancer symptoms. These anecdotal accounts gained traction, leading some researchers to take a closer look at whether this commonly used dewormer might hold hidden potential in oncology.

Ivermectin: A Nobel Prize-Winning Discovery

Unlike fenbendazole, ivermectin has played a well-established role in human medicine for decades. Originally derived from a natural compound found in soil bacteria, ivermectin became a revolutionary treatment for parasitic diseases, most notably river blindness and lymphatic filariasis. Its discovery and subsequent impact were so significant that the scientists behind it were awarded the Nobel Prize in Physiology or Medicine in 2015.

Ivermectin's introduction changed global health, particularly in regions where parasitic infections were widespread. It has been credited with saving millions of lives and improving the quality of life for countless individuals who would otherwise have suffered from debilitating parasitic diseases. Over time, its uses expanded to include treatments for scabies, lice, and other conditions, reinforcing its reputation as a safe and effective medication.

However, as with fenbendazole, ivermectin's story took an unexpected turn when researchers and independent investigators began noticing that it might have effects beyond treating parasites. Some laboratory studies indicated that ivermectin had properties that could interfere with cancer cell growth, leading to increased interest in its potential repurposing. While mainstream medical research has been slow to adopt this idea, the growing number of studies exploring ivermectin's mechanisms in cancer treatment suggests that it may be more than just an anti-parasitic drug.

The Search for Answers

The exploration of fenbendazole and ivermectin as cancer-fighting agents represents a growing trend in medicine: the repurposing of existing drugs for new therapeutic uses. Some of the most well-known treatments today started as medications for entirely different conditions. For example, metformin, a common diabetes drug, has been widely studied for its potential anti-cancer effects, and aspirin, originally a pain reliever, is now recognized for its role in heart disease prevention.

Given this history of repurposing medications, it is not unreasonable to investigate whether fenbendazole and ivermectin might have properties that could be beneficial in treating cancer. However, much of the discussion surrounding these drugs remains in the early stages. While preclinical research has begun to shed light on their potential mechanisms, there is still a long road ahead before definitive conclusions can be drawn.

What makes this topic so compelling is the fact that both drugs are inexpensive, widely available, and have established safety records. This makes them particularly intriguing for those seeking alternative or adjunctive cancer therapies, especially in cases where conventional treatments have been exhausted or have produced limited results.

As research continues and more people experiment with these drugs, the hope is that greater scientific scrutiny will bring clarity to their role in cancer treatment. Whether they turn out to be effective therapies or simply another case of misplaced optimism, their growing presence in the conversation about cancer care cannot be ignored.

A Long History of Safe Use

One of the most important aspects of both fenbendazole and ivermectin is their long-standing safety profiles. Unlike experimental drugs that require years of rigorous testing before being considered safe, these medications have been used for decades in their respective fields with minimal side effects. This history of use gives them a significant advantage when considering their potential repurposing for cancer treatment.

Fenbendazole has been a staple in veterinary medicine since its introduction in the 1970s. It belongs to the benzimidazole class of drugs, which are known for their ability to disrupt parasitic cells without harming the host. Farmers, veterinarians, and pet owners have relied on it to eliminate intestinal worms in a wide range of animals, from cattle and horses to household pets like dogs and cats. Its broad-spectrum activity and minimal toxicity have made it one of the most commonly used dewormers worldwide.

In the case of ivermectin, its impact has been even more far-reaching. After its discovery in the late 1970s, ivermectin quickly became a cornerstone in the fight against parasitic diseases in humans. It has been used to treat river blindness (onchocerciasis), lymphatic filariasis, and other neglected tropical diseases, particularly in regions where access to healthcare is limited. The drug's safety and effectiveness were so profound that in 2015, its discoverers were awarded the Nobel Prize in Physiology or Medicine.

Both drugs have been administered to millions of individuals and animals over the years, demonstrating consistent safety with relatively few adverse effects. When used at standard doses, they have well-documented tolerability, making them promising candidates for repurposing.

Regulatory Approval and Accessibility

One of the most intriguing aspects of fenbendazole and ivermectin is their widespread availability. Unlike many specialized cancer treatments that require prescriptions and are often expensive, these drugs are accessible and affordable.

Fenbendazole is available over the counter as a veterinary medication and can be purchased from feed stores, pet supply shops, and online retailers. While it is technically not approved for human use, some individuals have taken it upon themselves to experiment with it off-label, driven by anecdotal reports of its potential benefits in cancer treatment.

Ivermectin, on the other hand, is both a veterinary and human medication. It is approved by the FDA and the World Health Organization for treating parasitic infections in humans, and it is included on the WHO's List of Essential Medicines. As a result, it is widely available in pharmacies and through medical providers, particularly in countries where parasitic diseases are common.

The affordability of both drugs is another factor fueling interest in their potential role in cancer treatment. Traditional cancer therapies, such as chemotherapy and targeted drugs, can be prohibitively expensive, placing financial strain on patients and their families. In contrast, fenbendazole and ivermectin cost only a fraction of what conventional treatments do, making them an attractive option for those seeking alternative or supplementary therapies.

This accessibility, however, also presents challenges. Since neither drug is officially approved for cancer treatment, individuals who choose to use them must navigate their own dosing, safety considerations, and potential interactions with other treatments. Without medical oversight, there is a risk of improper usage, which underscores the need for more formal research and clinical trials to establish clear guidelines.

The question remains: Could these inexpensive, widely available drugs truly offer a new avenue for cancer treatment? As interest grows and research advances, the answers may soon become clearer.

The First Whispers of a Cancer Connection

For decades, fenbendazole and ivermectin were known purely as anti-parasitic medications. They were staples in veterinary and human medicine, respectively, with well-documented safety records. But in recent years, whispers of their potential as cancer treatments began surfacing in unexpected places—alternative health forums, anecdotal patient stories, and small-scale independent research.

The first reports were scattered. Individuals battling aggressive or late-stage cancers shared their experiences online, claiming that after taking fenbendazole or ivermectin, their tumors shrank or their disease stabilized. Some had originally been prescribed these medications for unrelated parasitic infections and noticed unexpected improvements in their cancer symptoms. Others intentionally sought them out after hearing of similar cases. These stories were difficult to verify, but they shared a common theme: patients who had exhausted conventional treatment options were looking elsewhere for hope.

The case that brought fenbendazole into the public eye was that of Joe Tippens, an American businessman who was diagnosed with terminal lung cancer. Facing a grim prognosis, Tippens decided to try fenbendazole after learning about its potential anti-cancer effects from a veterinarian. He combined it with a regimen of vitamins and supplements and, against the odds, experienced a remarkable recovery. His story spread rapidly, sparking interest in whether this widely used dewormer might hold real promise in oncology.

Ivermectin's cancer connection gained traction in a similar fashion. Some researchers had already been investigating its potential antiviral and anti-inflammatory properties, and along the way, they noticed its surprising effects on cancer cells in lab studies. As with fenbendazole, early anecdotal reports from patients began surfacing, further fueling interest. Unlike fenbendazole, which had no official human medical use, ivermectin already had an established place in human medicine, making it easier for individuals to access and experiment with.

Scientific Curiosity and Early Investigations

While early reports were largely anecdotal, the growing curiosity surrounding these drugs eventually caught the attention of the scientific community. Some researchers began exploring their potential mechanisms, questioning whether their effects on parasites could extend to cancer cells.

One of the most intriguing aspects was the way both drugs appeared to disrupt key biological processes essential for cancer growth. Fenbendazole, for instance, was found to interfere with microtubules—structures within cells that are critical for cell division. Some chemotherapy drugs work in a similar way, raising the possibility that fenbendazole might have unintentional anti-cancer properties.

Ivermectin, meanwhile, demonstrated the ability to influence cancer metabolism, suppress inflammation, and even trigger apoptosis, or programmed cell death, in certain cancer cell lines. Laboratory studies showed that it might be able to slow tumor progression, particularly in aggressive cancers resistant to conventional treatments.

At this stage, research remained limited, and skepticism within the medical community was high. The idea that two inexpensive, readily available drugs could have overlooked anti-cancer properties was met with resistance. Many experts cautioned that anecdotal reports were not enough and that rigorous clinical trials were needed before drawing any conclusions.

Despite these challenges, the momentum behind investigating fenbendazole and ivermectin for cancer continued to build. Small studies, case reports, and independent experiments added fuel to the fire, creating a growing movement of patients and researchers eager to see where the evidence would lead.

The Shift to Cancer Research

As the anecdotal stories surrounding fenbendazole and ivermectin continued to circulate, curiosity in the scientific community began to shift. Researchers who had previously focused on parasitic diseases started exploring the unexpected possibility that these drugs could have broader therapeutic benefits. While the idea of repurposing drugs was not new, the growing body of patient reports and preliminary studies began to warrant a more serious investigation into their potential role in cancer treatment.

One of the key factors driving this transition was the growing recognition that cancer cells share certain biological features with parasites. Both require a supply of nutrients, primarily glucose, to fuel their rapid growth. Additionally, cancer cells often rely on altered cellular processes to divide uncontrollably and evade the body's immune system. This similarity in metabolic demands and cell survival strategies created a theoretical link between the way these drugs target parasites and the way they might affect cancer cells.

In 2019, a study published in *Scientific Reports* examined the effects of ivermectin on various cancer cell lines. The researchers discovered that ivermectin interfered with the metabolic pathways that cancer cells rely on, slowing their growth and even triggering cell death in some instances. This was an exciting discovery, suggesting that ivermectin might be capable of modulating critical processes in cancer cells, similar to how it works to eliminate parasitic infections. However, the study was small, and its findings needed to be replicated to confirm its validity.

Similarly, research on fenbendazole showed promising results in preclinical models. In one animal study, researchers found that fenbendazole could inhibit tumor growth in mice, particularly in lung cancer. This effect appeared to be related to fenbendazole's ability to disrupt microtubules, which are essential for cell division. By interfering with the normal functioning of microtubules, fenbendazole could potentially stop cancer cells from dividing, much like chemotherapy drugs that target the same cellular structures.

As these preliminary findings emerged, researchers began to explore ways to incorporate fenbendazole and ivermectin into cancer treatment protocols, either alone or in combination with conventional therapies. The hope was that these drugs might act as adjuncts to enhance the effects of chemotherapy or immunotherapy, potentially improving patient outcomes and reducing the side effects associated with traditional treatments.

While scientific interest was growing, there were still many challenges to overcome. Both drugs had primarily been used to treat parasitic infections, not cancer, and their exact mechanisms of action in cancer cells were not well understood. More rigorous clinical trials would be needed to determine the appropriate dosages, treatment regimens, and potential interactions with other medications.

Nonetheless, the shift toward cancer research marked an exciting turning point in the story of fenbendazole and ivermectin. As more studies are conducted and evidence begins to accumulate, we may find that these once overlooked drugs hold untapped potential in the fight against cancer. The growing interest in repurposing existing drugs for cancer treatment is a reminder that the path to new therapies is often unexpected and, at times, surprising.

Chapter 2: How Fenbendazole and Ivermectin Work Against Cancer

Cutting Off Cancer's Energy Supply

Cancer cells behave differently from normal cells, growing and dividing at an accelerated rate while finding ways to resist the body's natural defenses. One of the key factors driving their survival is an insatiable demand for energy. Unlike healthy cells, which can switch between different fuel sources, cancer cells rely heavily on glucose metabolism to sustain their rapid growth. This process, known as the Warburg effect, allows cancer cells to generate energy even in environments with low oxygen, giving them a survival advantage.

Both fenbendazole and ivermectin appear to disrupt this metabolic process in ways that could weaken cancer cells and make them more vulnerable to treatment. Studies suggest that these drugs interfere with glucose uptake, essentially starving tumors of the fuel they need to grow. By cutting off this energy supply, cancer cells struggle to maintain their function, leading to slower growth and, in some cases, cell death.

Ivermectin, in particular, has been shown to affect mitochondrial function—the energy-producing structures within cells. In laboratory studies, it has demonstrated the ability to disrupt cancer cell metabolism, making it more difficult for tumors to generate energy efficiently. Without a steady supply of fuel, cancer cells lose their ability to divide rapidly, and their survival mechanisms begin to break down.

Fenbendazole's effects on cancer metabolism are slightly different but equally promising. In addition to interfering with glucose metabolism, it has been shown to limit the ability of cancer cells to utilize certain proteins essential for their survival. This dual action makes it an intriguing candidate for combination therapy, as it may work alongside other treatments to increase effectiveness.

Cancer's Weak Spot

What makes these findings especially compelling is that cancer cells, unlike normal cells, are often highly dependent on specific survival pathways. While healthy cells can adapt to changes in energy availability, cancer cells tend to be more rigid, making them vulnerable to disruptions in their metabolic processes. This is why some of the most successful cancer treatments target the ways tumors obtain energy and nutrients.

By interfering with these processes, fenbendazole and ivermectin could provide a new angle for weakening tumors and slowing disease progression. The research is still in its early stages, but the concept of targeting cancer metabolism is not new. Many conventional treatments, including chemotherapy and targeted therapies, aim to exploit these vulnerabilities. If further studies confirm that these inexpensive, widely available drugs can achieve similar effects, they could represent a significant breakthrough in cancer treatment strategies.

Although much remains to be learned about the precise mechanisms behind their effects, the growing body of research suggests that these medications have potential far beyond their original uses. The next step in the investigation is understanding how they interact with cancer cells at a deeper level and determining the best ways to integrate them into broader treatment plans.

Disrupting Cancer Cell Division

One of the defining traits of cancer is uncontrolled cell division. Unlike normal cells, which follow a regulated cycle of growth and death, cancer cells multiply relentlessly, forming tumors and spreading to other parts of the body. This ability to divide rapidly is largely dependent on structures called microtubules, which act like scaffolding within cells, guiding them through the process of replication.

Fenbendazole appears to interfere with these microtubules in a way similar to some well-known chemotherapy drugs. In laboratory studies, researchers have found that fenbendazole binds to microtubule proteins, preventing them from assembling properly. Without functional microtubules, cancer cells struggle to complete the process of division, ultimately leading to their death. This disruption is particularly effective against fast-growing tumors, which rely heavily on constant cell replication to sustain themselves.

The key difference between fenbendazole and traditional chemotherapy is its lower toxicity. Many chemotherapy drugs that target microtubules, such as paclitaxel and vinblastine, are associated with severe side effects, including damage to healthy dividing cells in the bone marrow and digestive system. Fenbendazole, on the other hand, has been used in animals for decades with an excellent safety record, suggesting that it may offer a gentler approach to interfering with cancer growth.

Ivermectin's Role in Stopping Cancer's Spread

Ivermectin operates differently from fenbendazole but may complement its effects. Instead of targeting microtubules, ivermectin appears to interfere with several signaling pathways that cancer cells use to communicate and spread.

One of these pathways involves a process called epithelial-to-mesenchymal transition (EMT), which allows cancer cells to become more mobile. In many cancers, EMT is what enables tumors to invade nearby tissues and spread to distant organs. Studies have shown that ivermectin can suppress EMT, effectively limiting the ability of cancer cells to migrate.

Additionally, ivermectin has demonstrated the ability to increase the sensitivity of cancer cells to existing treatments. Some researchers have explored its use alongside chemotherapy, where it has been shown to enhance the effects of traditional drugs by weakening cancer cells' defenses. This suggests that ivermectin could be particularly useful in combination therapy, helping to reduce drug resistance and improve overall outcomes.

While these findings are promising, much of the research remains in the early stages. However, the fact that both fenbendazole and ivermectin can disrupt cancer's ability to grow and spread through different mechanisms makes them particularly interesting candidates for further study. If their effects can be validated in clinical trials, they may provide a new, low-cost option for patients seeking alternative or complementary cancer treatments.

Triggering Cancer Cell Death: Apoptosis and Autophagy

One of the most important strategies in cancer treatment is finding ways to make cancer cells destroy themselves. Unlike healthy cells, which have built-in mechanisms to regulate their lifespan, cancer cells resist normal signals for cell death, allowing them to multiply uncontrollably. This is where fenbendazole and ivermectin show intriguing potential—both have been found to encourage processes that force cancer cells to self-destruct.

Apoptosis, also known as programmed cell death, is a natural process that removes damaged or unnecessary cells from the body. Many cancer treatments, including chemotherapy and targeted therapies, aim to reactivate apoptosis in tumors that have learned to evade this process. Research suggests that ivermectin can increase apoptosis in certain types of cancer cells, effectively restoring their ability to die when they become damaged or abnormal.

Fenbendazole also appears to promote apoptosis, but it may do so in a different way. Studies indicate that it interferes with proteins that cancer cells rely on to avoid cell death, making them more susceptible to destruction. By reactivating this natural fail-safe mechanism, fenbendazole may help shrink tumors and prevent cancer from spreading.

Another process linked to cancer cell death is autophagy. This is the body's way of recycling damaged or unnecessary components within cells. In normal circumstances, autophagy helps maintain cellular health, but in cancer cells, it can be hijacked to support their survival. Interestingly, ivermectin has been found to disrupt this balance, pushing cancer cells toward excessive autophagy, which ultimately leads to their destruction. Some researchers believe that this could be a major factor in its potential anti-cancer effects.

Why Cancer Cells Are Vulnerable to These Effects

The reason fenbendazole and ivermectin can affect cancer cells while leaving healthy cells relatively unharmed is rooted in the way cancer cells behave. Unlike normal cells, which are flexible and adaptive, cancer cells often depend on very specific survival pathways. Once a tumor finds a way to keep itself alive, it becomes heavily reliant on that mechanism. This creates a unique vulnerability—if you take away its survival crutch, the cancer cell collapses.

For example, some cancers become completely dependent on certain proteins that prevent apoptosis. If a drug like fenbendazole disrupts those proteins, the cancer cell has no backup plan and dies off. Similarly, cancer cells often rely on high levels of autophagy to maintain their energy needs. If ivermectin forces them into excessive autophagy, they essentially consume themselves from the inside out.

This selective pressure is what makes drug repurposing so interesting. Many existing medications have effects on biological pathways that were never originally explored for cancer. In the case of fenbendazole and ivermectin, their ability to push cancer cells toward self-destruction—without causing significant harm to normal cells—makes them promising candidates for further study.

While much of this research is still in its early stages, the results so far suggest that these drugs may offer an effective way to weaken tumors and increase their vulnerability to other treatments. Their ability to trigger apoptosis and disrupt autophagy adds another layer to their potential as part of a multi-faceted cancer treatment approach.

The Role of Inflammation and the Immune System

Cancer thrives in an environment of chronic inflammation. Unlike normal tissue, which repairs itself after injury and returns to a balanced state, cancerous growths manipulate inflammatory pathways to sustain their survival. Inflammation provides cancer cells with the growth factors they need to multiply, weakens immune responses, and creates an ideal setting for tumors to spread. This is why many modern cancer treatments aim to control inflammation as part of an overall strategy to fight the disease.

Ivermectin has drawn attention for its ability to regulate inflammation in ways that may be beneficial in cancer treatment. Researchers have found that it suppresses the activity of certain inflammatory proteins that fuel tumor progression. By reducing this inflammation, ivermectin may help slow the growth of tumors and make them more vulnerable to attack by the immune system.

Fenbendazole, on the other hand, appears to have indirect effects on inflammation through its impact on oxidative stress. Oxidative stress occurs when there is an imbalance between harmful free radicals and the body's ability to neutralize them. Cancer cells often use oxidative stress to their advantage, but fenbendazole has been shown to interfere with this process, potentially making it harder for tumors to survive.

Strengthening the Body's Natural Defenses

A well-functioning immune system is one of the best defenses against cancer. The body has specialized cells, such as T-cells and natural killer cells, that are designed to seek out and destroy abnormal cells before they can become dangerous. However, cancer often finds ways to evade this immune surveillance, creating a kind of invisibility cloak that allows tumors to grow unchecked.

Ivermectin has been found to enhance immune activity in ways that may help counteract this problem. Some studies suggest that it can boost the effectiveness of immune cells, making them more aggressive in targeting cancer. It may also increase the visibility of cancer cells, making it easier for the immune system to recognize and eliminate them.

Fenbendazole's potential role in immune support is less well understood, but some early research suggests that it could have indirect benefits. By weakening cancer cells and disrupting their ability to grow, it may create conditions that allow the immune system to regain control.

The relationship between these drugs, inflammation, and immune function is still an area of active investigation, but the findings so far suggest that they may work in multiple ways to weaken cancer's hold on the body. If these effects can be further validated in human studies, they could represent a powerful new approach to cancer treatment—

one that not only targets tumors directly but also strengthens the body's ability to fight back.

Preventing Tumor Growth and Metastasis

One of the most dangerous aspects of cancer is its ability to spread beyond its original location. While some cancers remain localized, many develop the ability to invade nearby tissues and travel to distant organs—a process known as metastasis. Once cancer spreads, treatment becomes significantly more challenging, and survival rates drop. This is why researchers are constantly searching for ways to stop cancer from metastasizing, and it appears that both fenbendazole and ivermectin may play a role in this effort.

Ivermectin has been studied for its ability to interfere with signaling pathways that cancer cells use to move and invade new tissues. One of the ways it does this is by blocking the epithelial-to-mesenchymal transition (EMT), a process that makes cancer cells more mobile. In aggressive cancers, EMT allows tumor cells to detach, travel through the bloodstream, and establish new tumors in distant organs. By suppressing EMT, ivermectin may help keep cancer contained, reducing the likelihood of metastasis.

Fenbendazole, though primarily known for its effects on microtubules, also appears to impact cancer's ability to spread. Some research suggests that it weakens cancer cells' structural integrity, making it more difficult for them to break free and migrate. Additionally, since it disrupts the cellular skeleton, cancer cells may struggle to move efficiently, further reducing their ability to invade new areas.

Starving Tumors of Their Blood Supply

For a tumor to grow beyond a certain size, it must create its own blood supply—a process called angiogenesis. This allows it to receive oxygen and nutrients, fueling its expansion. Many conventional cancer drugs target angiogenesis to choke off a tumor's resources, and there is evidence that ivermectin may have a similar effect.

Ivermectin has been found to inhibit key growth factors that tumors use to signal the formation of new blood vessels. Without these signals, tumors struggle to develop the vascular networks they need, slowing their progression. This is particularly important in aggressive cancers that rely heavily on rapid blood vessel formation.

Fenbendazole's potential effects on angiogenesis are not as well studied, but its role in disrupting cellular function may contribute indirectly. By interfering with cancer cell metabolism and division, it may reduce the energy and signaling power tumors need to sustain angiogenesis, making it harder for them to continue expanding.

These combined effects—blocking metastasis, preventing tumor movement, and limiting blood vessel growth—suggest that these drugs may not only weaken existing tumors but also help prevent new ones from taking hold. While much more research is needed to confirm these effects in humans, the early findings provide strong motivation for further study. If these mechanisms can be harnessed effectively, they could provide a new, affordable tool for keeping cancer from spreading and making it easier to control with other therapies.

Chapter 3: Reviewing the Scientific Studies and Evidence

What the Research Says About Fenbendazole

While fenbendazole's reputation as a potential cancer treatment largely stems from anecdotal reports, scientific research has begun to investigate its mechanisms and effectiveness in cancer therapy. Most of the studies conducted so far have been in laboratory settings or animal models, but the findings have been promising enough to warrant further investigation.

One of the earliest pieces of research linking fenbendazole to cancer treatment was a study published in 2008 that examined its effects on non-small cell lung cancer cells. The researchers found that fenbendazole disrupted the cancer cells' ability to divide by targeting their microtubules—the same structures affected by certain chemotherapy drugs. By interfering with these structures, fenbendazole prevented the cells from completing their normal cycle of replication, leading to cell death.

Another study, published in *Scientific Reports* in 2018, explored fenbendazole's ability to inhibit tumor growth in mice. The results showed that mice treated with fenbendazole had significantly slower tumor progression compared to untreated controls. The researchers proposed that this effect was likely due to fenbendazole's ability to impair glucose metabolism, cutting off the fuel supply that cancer cells depend on for survival.

Combining Fenbendazole with Other Treatments

One of the more interesting aspects of fenbendazole research is its potential to work alongside other cancer treatments. Some studies have examined how it interacts with chemotherapy and radiation, and the results suggest that it may enhance their effectiveness.

In one experiment, researchers tested fenbendazole in combination with radiation therapy on lung cancer cells. They found that fenbendazole made the cells more sensitive to radiation, leading to greater levels of cell death. This suggests that fenbendazole may act as a radiosensitizer, meaning it makes cancer cells more vulnerable to radiation damage while sparing healthy cells.

Similarly, studies have indicated that fenbendazole may enhance the effects of certain chemotherapy drugs. By weakening cancer cells and disrupting their ability to recover from treatment, fenbendazole could help prevent tumors from developing resistance to conventional therapies.

While these studies are promising, it is important to note that human clinical trials are still lacking. Most of the existing research has been conducted in cell cultures and animal models, which, while useful, do not always translate directly to human treatment. However, the evidence so far suggests that fenbendazole is worth further study as a potential adjunct to existing cancer therapies.

As interest in drug repurposing continues to grow, more researchers are turning their attention to fenbendazole's effects on different types of cancer. The next step will be conducting controlled clinical trials to determine how it works in human patients, what doses are effective, and whether it can be safely integrated into existing treatment protocols.

What the Research Says About Ivermectin

While ivermectin is best known for its role in treating parasitic infections, research over the past decade has revealed surprising anti-cancer properties. Laboratory studies have shown that ivermectin can interfere with multiple processes that cancer cells rely on, including cell division, metabolism, and immune system evasion. These findings have led to growing interest in repurposing ivermectin as a potential cancer treatment, though human clinical trials remain limited.

One of the most cited studies on ivermectin's anti-cancer effects was published in *EMBO Molecular Medicine* in 2017. The research found that ivermectin could inhibit the growth of multiple types of cancer cells, including breast, ovarian, and glioblastoma (a highly aggressive brain cancer). The study suggested that ivermectin works by disrupting cancer cell metabolism, making it harder for tumors to generate the energy they need to survive.

Another study, published in *Frontiers in Pharmacology* in 2020, explored ivermectin's ability to block cancer cell signaling pathways. Researchers found that ivermectin could interfere with Wnt signaling—a process that many cancers exploit to grow and spread. By disrupting this pathway, ivermectin made it more difficult for cancer cells to divide, effectively slowing tumor progression.

Ivermectin's Potential in Drug-Resistant Cancers

One of the most exciting areas of ivermectin research is its potential role in overcoming drug resistance. Many cancers develop resistance to chemotherapy over time, making treatment less effective. Some studies have suggested that ivermectin may help reverse this resistance, restoring the effectiveness of traditional cancer drugs.

A 2018 study published in *Biochemical and Biophysical Research Communications* found that ivermectin increased the sensitivity of drug-resistant leukemia cells to chemotherapy. The researchers concluded that ivermectin might work by disrupting cancer cells' ability to pump out chemotherapy drugs, allowing the treatment to remain inside the cells long enough to take effect.

Similarly, a 2021 study in *Cancer Chemotherapy and Pharmacology* suggested that ivermectin could enhance the effectiveness of doxorubicin, a widely used chemotherapy drug. By interfering with the cancer cells' defense mechanisms, ivermectin appeared to make the chemotherapy more potent.

Although these findings are promising, most studies on ivermectin's anti-cancer properties have been conducted in cell cultures and animal models. More research is needed to determine whether these effects translate to human patients, particularly in terms of safe dosing and potential side effects. However, given its affordability, established safety profile, and broad mechanism of action, ivermectin remains a strong candidate for further study as part of a multi-faceted cancer treatment approach.

Case Studies and Anecdotal Evidence

While laboratory research has begun to uncover the mechanisms by which fenbendazole and ivermectin may affect cancer cells, much of the current interest in these drugs comes from anecdotal reports—real-world stories of patients who have used them as part of their treatment plan. These case studies, though not scientific proof on their own, have drawn attention to the possibility that these medications may have benefits beyond their original uses.

One of the most well-known cases is that of **Joe Tippens**, an American businessman who was diagnosed with stage 4 small cell lung cancer. His doctors had given him just a few months to live, and after exhausting conventional treatment options, he turned to fenbendazole based on a recommendation from a veterinarian. Alongside a regimen of supplements, he began taking fenbendazole daily. To the surprise of his medical team, follow-up scans showed that his tumors had shrunk, and within months, they were gone. Tippens' story spread widely, inspiring others in similar situations to try fenbendazole.

Other patients have shared similar experiences, particularly those with aggressive or treatment-resistant cancers. Some have reported tumor shrinkage or slowed progression after incorporating fenbendazole into their treatment regimen. While these reports are encouraging, they also highlight the need for controlled clinical trials to determine whether the effects observed are due to the medication itself or other factors.

Ivermectin's Growing Reputation

Ivermectin has also gained attention due to anecdotal reports of its potential effectiveness against cancer. In online forums and patient support groups, individuals with various types of cancer have claimed that taking ivermectin—sometimes in combination with conventional therapies—has led to improvements in their condition.

A case report published in *Medicina* in 2022 described a patient with stage 4 colon cancer who saw unexpected improvements after adding ivermectin to his treatment. His tumors, which had been progressing despite standard therapies, showed signs of regression. While this was only a single case, it added to the growing body of reports suggesting that ivermectin may have unrecognized potential in oncology.

Physicians in integrative and alternative medicine circles have also begun to experiment with off-label ivermectin use for cancer patients, often combining it with repurposed drugs like doxycycline, metformin, and statins. Some practitioners believe that ivermectin's ability to enhance immune function and inhibit tumor growth makes it a valuable addition to multi-drug protocols.

While these stories are compelling, they do not replace rigorous scientific studies. Anecdotal evidence is often subject to bias, placebo effects, and other variables that make it difficult to draw firm conclusions. However, the sheer volume of patient reports has prompted some researchers to take these drugs more seriously, leading to more studies aimed at determining whether fenbendazole and ivermectin truly have anti-cancer properties.

As more data emerges, the hope is that anecdotal reports will be supplemented with concrete scientific evidence, providing clarity on the real potential of these drugs in cancer treatment.

Current and Past Clinical Trials

Despite the growing interest in fenbendazole and ivermectin as potential cancer treatments, clinical trials investigating their effectiveness remain limited. However, some studies have begun to emerge, providing a more structured look at how these drugs interact with cancer cells in human patients.

One of the most notable clinical trials exploring ivermectin's role in cancer treatment was conducted on **triple-negative breast cancer**, an aggressive form of the disease with limited treatment options. Researchers at the University of Texas found that ivermectin significantly slowed the growth of cancer cells in lab settings and animal models. The study prompted discussions about whether ivermectin could be repurposed for human use, leading to a **Phase 1 clinical trial** to evaluate its safety and effectiveness in cancer patients.

Additionally, a **2021 study published in Frontiers in Pharmacology** reviewed multiple small-scale trials and case reports on ivermectin's anti-cancer properties. The researchers concluded that while preclinical evidence was promising, larger and more controlled trials were needed to determine its true impact.

Fenbendazole, in contrast, has yet to receive the same level of clinical investigation. While animal studies have demonstrated its ability to suppress tumor growth, no large-scale human trials have been conducted. Some researchers have speculated that since fenbendazole is a veterinary drug, securing funding for human trials has been a challenge. Pharmaceutical companies are often reluctant to invest in clinical trials for non-patentable, low-cost medications, making it difficult for drugs like fenbendazole to receive mainstream scientific validation.

The Challenge of Moving from Lab Research to Human Studies

One of the biggest hurdles in evaluating repurposed drugs for cancer is the transition from laboratory research to human trials. In cell cultures and animal models, both fenbendazole and ivermectin have shown the ability to slow tumor growth, interfere with cancer metabolism, and even enhance the effects of chemotherapy. However, human biology is more complex, and what works in a petri dish does not always translate to real-world clinical success.

Regulatory challenges also slow down the process. Unlike new drug candidates developed by pharmaceutical companies, repurposed drugs like fenbendazole and ivermectin often lack the financial backing needed to conduct large, multi-phase clinical trials. This means that much of the existing evidence remains stuck at the preclinical stage, leaving patients to rely on anecdotal reports and self-experimentation.

Despite these challenges, interest in conducting trials continues to grow. Independent researchers and patient advocacy groups have pushed for more funding and attention, hoping that formal studies will eventually provide clearer answers. Some smaller studies are underway, particularly in regions where access to expensive cancer treatments is limited, and ivermectin is already widely available.

The hope is that with more research, these drugs will either be confirmed as viable cancer treatments or ruled out based on scientific evidence. Until then, the conversation around repurposing fenbendazole and ivermectin for cancer remains a mix of promising discoveries, patient-led experimentation, and the need for more rigorous clinical validation.

Limitations and Future Research Needs

While the evidence surrounding fenbendazole and ivermectin as potential cancer treatments is compelling, significant gaps remain. Much of the research conducted so far has been in laboratory settings or animal models, with only a handful of small-scale human case reports and trials. Without large, well-designed clinical studies, it is difficult to determine exactly how effective these drugs are in human patients, what the optimal dosages might be, and whether they work best alone or in combination with other therapies.

One of the key challenges in studying these drugs is the lack of financial incentive for pharmaceutical companies. Since both fenbendazole and ivermectin are inexpensive and already widely available, there is little commercial motivation to fund expensive clinical trials. Most drug development is driven by profit potential, and repurposing old drugs does not generate the same return on investment as developing new, patentable treatments. As a result, much of the research has been driven by independent scientists, universities, and patient-led initiatives rather than major pharmaceutical companies.

Addressing Safety and Dosage Concerns

Although fenbendazole and ivermectin have well-established safety profiles in their traditional uses, their long-term effects in cancer treatment remain unknown. The dosages required to achieve anti-cancer effects may differ from those used for parasitic infections, raising questions about potential side effects, toxicity, and drug interactions.

For example, while ivermectin is considered safe at standard doses, high doses may cause neurological side effects, including dizziness and confusion. Similarly, fenbendazole is well tolerated in animals, but its effects in humans have not been thoroughly studied. Patients experimenting with these drugs often rely on anecdotal dosing guidelines, which may not always be optimal or safe.

Another important consideration is how these drugs interact with conventional cancer treatments. Some studies suggest that they may enhance the effects of chemotherapy and radiation, while others warn that they could interfere with certain drugs. Without more research, it remains unclear how best to integrate them into existing cancer treatment protocols.

The Path Forward

Despite these limitations, the interest in repurposing fenbendazole and ivermectin for cancer treatment is growing. More researchers are recognizing the need for clinical trials, and patient advocacy groups are pushing for further study. If these drugs prove to be effective, they could offer a low-cost, accessible option for cancer patients, particularly in regions where conventional treatments are unaffordable or unavailable.

Until then, the best approach is cautious optimism. While the early findings are promising, they are not a substitute for proven cancer treatments. Patients considering these drugs should do so under the guidance of a knowledgeable healthcare professional, and researchers must continue working toward the larger studies needed to confirm their potential benefits. If ongoing investigations provide more concrete evidence, fenbendazole and ivermectin could one day become important tools in the fight against cancer.

Chapter 4: Setting Up a Fenbendazole or Ivermectin Protocol

Dosing Strategies for Fenbendazole

Fenbendazole was never designed for human consumption, so there is no officially recommended dosage for cancer treatment. However, people who have experimented with it off-label have reported using it in relatively consistent ways, following protocols inspired by veterinary dosages and early anecdotal cases.

One of the most widely known regimens comes from Joe Tippens, the businessman who popularized fenbendazole as a potential cancer treatment. His approach involved taking **222 mg of fenbendazole (one packet of Panacur C, a common brand) per day for three days, followed by four days off**, repeating this cycle indefinitely. This "three days on, four days off" method was initially derived from its use in animals and was intended to minimize any potential toxicity or side effects.

Some individuals choose to take fenbendazole continuously without breaks, particularly those with more aggressive or late-stage cancers. Others have experimented with alternating dosing schedules, adjusting based on their response. The lack of clinical trials means that these protocols are largely experimental, and individuals often tweak their approach based on personal experience or consultation with integrative health practitioners.

Choosing the Right Form

Fenbendazole is most commonly available as a **powdered dewormer**, sold in small packets for dogs and other animals. While this is the form most widely used in anecdotal cancer protocols, some people opt for **capsules or compounded versions** to ensure more precise dosing.

The powdered form is typically mixed into food or a beverage to improve absorption. Since fenbendazole is fat-soluble, some users take it with a source of healthy fat, such as coconut oil or avocado, to enhance bioavailability. Others combine it with certain supplements thought to improve absorption or effectiveness, though research on this is still in its early stages.

Consistency Matters

For those who have reported success with fenbendazole, consistency appears to be a key factor. Many individuals emphasize the importance of **sticking to the protocol long-term**, rather than expecting immediate results. Some claim to have seen changes in their cancer markers within weeks, while others report improvements only after several months of use.

Because there is no standardized medical guidance for using fenbendazole in cancer, it is crucial for individuals to **monitor their health closely** and, where possible, work with a healthcare professional who is open to exploring repurposed drug approaches. Tracking symptoms, tumor markers, and imaging results can help guide adjustments to the protocol over time.

Although more research is needed, the existing reports suggest that fenbendazole may be a useful tool in a broader cancer treatment plan. However, as with any experimental therapy, its use should be approached with careful consideration and ongoing evaluation.

Dosing Strategies for Ivermectin

Ivermectin has been widely used in human medicine for decades, making its dosing guidelines more established than those for fenbendazole. However, its potential application in cancer treatment is still emerging, and most of the available dosing protocols come from off-label use and experimental research rather than formal medical recommendations.

One of the most referenced dosing strategies comes from researchers studying ivermectin's anti-cancer properties. A commonly cited regimen suggests a dosage of **0.2 to 0.4 mg per kilogram of body weight**, taken daily or in cycles, depending on the individual's response. For a person weighing 70 kg (154 lbs), this would amount to **14 to 28 mg per day**. Some individuals take it continuously, while others follow a pulse-dosing schedule, such as **five days on, two days off** or alternating weeks.

Some protocols recommend taking ivermectin in the evening, as it is absorbed more effectively when taken with food. Since it is fat-soluble, pairing it with a meal containing healthy fats can enhance its absorption, potentially improving its effectiveness.

Formulations and Delivery Methods

Ivermectin is available in several forms, including **tablets, liquid solutions, and topical formulations**. The **tablet form** is the most commonly used in human medicine and is the preferred option for off-label cancer treatment due to its precise dosing and ease of administration.

Veterinary formulations, such as **liquid ivermectin** intended for livestock, are also widely available and sometimes used by those seeking cost-effective alternatives. However, these formulations often require careful dilution to achieve the correct dosage and should be used with caution. Some liquid versions contain additional inactive ingredients not meant for human consumption, making pharmaceutical-grade tablets the safest option when possible.

There has also been discussion about **combining ivermectin with other repurposed drugs** in cancer protocols. Some practitioners suggest that it works well alongside drugs like doxycycline, metformin, and statins, which have also been explored for their anti-cancer potential. The rationale behind this approach is that these medications may have synergistic effects, targeting cancer through multiple mechanisms at once.

Length of Use and Adjustments

Since ivermectin's role in cancer treatment is still being studied, there is no universal guideline on how long to take it. Some individuals have reported benefits after **weeks**

or months of consistent use, while others continue their regimen indefinitely as part of a long-term maintenance strategy.

Adjustments to dosing are often based on **symptom changes, tumor marker levels, or imaging results**. Some practitioners recommend starting at a lower dose and gradually increasing to assess tolerance, while others begin with a full dose from the start. As with any experimental treatment, it is essential for individuals using ivermectin off-label to monitor their health closely and seek professional guidance where possible.

While the research on ivermectin and cancer is still developing, its established safety profile, affordability, and accessibility make it a compelling candidate for further study. The challenge now is translating laboratory findings into structured clinical trials to determine the best dosing strategies, potential interactions, and long-term effects in cancer patients.

Combining with Other Supplements

While fenbendazole and ivermectin have shown potential as repurposed cancer treatments, many individuals using these drugs off-label incorporate additional supplements into their protocol to enhance effectiveness. Some of these supplements are believed to work synergistically, helping to improve absorption, support the immune system, or further weaken cancer cells. Although clinical data is still limited, anecdotal reports and emerging research suggest that certain supplements may play a beneficial role when combined with these medications.

One of the most commonly included supplements is **curcumin**, the active compound in turmeric. Curcumin has well-documented anti-inflammatory and anti-cancer properties, with studies suggesting that it can inhibit tumor growth, reduce angiogenesis (the formation of new blood vessels that feed tumors), and promote apoptosis in cancer cells. Some individuals take curcumin alongside fenbendazole or ivermectin, believing that it helps enhance their effects. Since curcumin is fat-soluble, it is often taken with a meal containing healthy fats or with black pepper extract (piperine) to improve absorption.

Another widely used supplement is **vitamin E**, particularly in its natural form as tocotrienols. Some research suggests that vitamin E can support apoptosis in cancer cells and improve the bioavailability of other compounds. Joe Tippens, the businessman who popularized fenbendazole as a cancer treatment, included vitamin E in his protocol, believing it played a role in his recovery. However, there is ongoing debate about whether high doses of certain forms of vitamin E might interfere with some cancer treatments, making it important to use with caution.

The Role of CBD and Other Natural Compounds

Cannabidiol (**CBD**) has also gained attention for its potential role in cancer treatment. Studies have suggested that CBD may help slow tumor growth, reduce inflammation, and enhance the effects of other therapies. Some people include CBD in their regimen alongside fenbendazole or ivermectin, believing that it may enhance their impact. Additionally, CBD is often used to help manage symptoms such as pain, nausea, and anxiety, which can be particularly beneficial for individuals undergoing conventional cancer treatments.

Other supplements frequently included in these regimens include:

Berberine, which has been studied for its ability to inhibit cancer cell metabolism and may work synergistically with ivermectin.
Quercetin, a flavonoid with anti-inflammatory and antioxidant properties that may help slow tumor progression.
Resveratrol, found in grapes and red wine, which has shown potential in enhancing apoptosis in certain cancers.
Omega-3 fatty acids, which may help modulate inflammation and support overall immune health.

While these supplements are often included based on anecdotal evidence, it is important to approach them with caution. Some supplements can interact with medications or have unintended effects when combined with specific cancer treatments. Individuals considering adding supplements to their protocol should research carefully and, where possible, consult with a healthcare professional familiar with integrative oncology.

The combination of fenbendazole, ivermectin, and supportive supplements represents an emerging area of interest in cancer treatment. While much of the evidence remains anecdotal, ongoing research may clarify how these compounds work together and whether they provide meaningful benefits in a structured treatment approach.

Side Effects and Safety Considerations

While fenbendazole and ivermectin have long-standing safety records in their original uses, taking them off-label for cancer treatment presents unique considerations.

Since neither drug has undergone large-scale clinical trials for cancer, most of the available safety data comes from their use in veterinary medicine or as antiparasitic treatments in humans. Understanding the potential risks and how to mitigate them is essential for those considering these drugs as part of a broader treatment plan.

Fenbendazole is generally well tolerated in animals, with few reported side effects even at higher doses. The most common issues observed in anecdotal human use include **mild digestive discomfort**, such as nausea, bloating, or diarrhea. These effects tend to subside as the body adjusts to the medication. Some individuals also report **fatigue** or a temporary increase in cancer-related symptoms, which may be due to a "die-off" effect as cancer cells weaken and release toxic byproducts. Drinking plenty of water and supporting liver function with antioxidants like N-acetylcysteine (NAC) or milk thistle may help mitigate this.

There is limited data on fenbendazole's long-term use in humans, which raises concerns about **unknown toxicity risks** with prolonged treatment. Since the drug was developed for short-term parasite elimination, its impact on human organs over extended periods remains uncertain. Some individuals cycle their usage—taking breaks to allow the body to reset—to minimize any potential risks.

Ivermectin's Safety Profile and Potential Risks

Ivermectin has been extensively studied in humans for its antiparasitic effects, and at standard doses, it is considered very safe. Millions of people worldwide have taken it to treat infections such as river blindness and scabies, with only minor side effects reported. However, when used at **higher doses or for extended periods**, some individuals experience neurological side effects, including **dizziness, brain fog, or temporary confusion**. These symptoms are thought to result from ivermectin's effect on certain neurotransmitter pathways.

Rare but serious reactions have been documented in individuals who have a genetic mutation affecting **P-glycoprotein**, a protein that helps regulate drug movement in the body. People with this mutation may be more susceptible to ivermectin toxicity, leading to more pronounced neurological effects. While this mutation is relatively uncommon, it highlights the importance of starting at a lower dose and monitoring for any adverse effects.

Additionally, ivermectin has been known to interact with **certain medications**, including blood thinners, immunosuppressants, and some chemotherapy drugs. Individuals taking multiple medications should carefully research potential interactions or consult with a knowledgeable healthcare provider.

Mitigating Side Effects and Ensuring Safe Use

For those considering using fenbendazole or ivermectin off-label, the following precautions may help improve safety and effectiveness:

- **Start with a lower dose and gradually increase** to assess tolerance.
- **Take with food, especially healthy fats,** to improve absorption and reduce gastrointestinal discomfort.
- **Support liver health** with supplements like NAC, milk thistle, or alpha-lipoic acid, particularly for those on long-term protocols.
- **Stay hydrated** to help flush toxins released from dying cancer cells.
- **Monitor for side effects** such as dizziness, nausea, or fatigue, and adjust dosing as needed.

Since no standardized medical guidelines exist for using these drugs in cancer treatment, those incorporating them into their regimen must be proactive in tracking their health and making informed decisions. While the overall safety profiles of fenbendazole and ivermectin are reassuring, further research is needed to fully understand the risks and best practices for long-term use in cancer patients.

Adjusting the Protocol Based on Response

Since fenbendazole and ivermectin are being used off-label for cancer treatment, there are no universal guidelines for how to adjust dosages over time. Instead, individuals who incorporate these drugs into their regimen often monitor their body's response and make changes accordingly. Tracking progress, recognizing early signs of effectiveness, and knowing when to modify dosing are essential components of a safe and effective protocol.

One of the first indicators that a protocol may be working is a change in **tumor markers**. Many cancers produce specific proteins that can be measured in the blood, such as CA-125 for ovarian cancer or PSA for prostate cancer. Regular testing can help determine whether a tumor is shrinking, stabilizing, or continuing to grow. Some individuals using fenbendazole or ivermectin have reported drops in their tumor marker levels after several weeks or months of consistent use. However, it is important to remember that changes in markers do not always correlate perfectly with tumor size or overall progression, so they should be interpreted alongside other clinical assessments.

Another way people monitor their progress is through **imaging scans**, such as MRIs, CT scans, or PET scans. While these tests are typically scheduled at longer intervals, they provide a clearer picture of how a tumor is responding to treatment. Some individuals who have used fenbendazole or ivermectin report a slowing of tumor growth or even partial shrinkage on follow-up scans, though this is highly variable and depends on many factors, including cancer type, stage, and overall treatment plan.

Recognizing When to Adjust Dosage

Adjustments to dosing are usually based on **symptom response and side effects**. Some individuals find that they tolerate their chosen dose well and continue with it indefinitely, while others notice side effects that may require modifications. Common reasons for adjusting a protocol include:

- **Increased fatigue or neurological symptoms** – Some people using ivermectin report brain fog or dizziness, particularly at higher doses. In these cases, reducing the dose or switching to an intermittent schedule (e.g., every other day) may help.
- **Gastrointestinal discomfort** – Fenbendazole can sometimes cause nausea or bloating, particularly when first starting. Lowering the dose and taking it with food can often alleviate this.
- **Lack of response after several months** – If there are no measurable changes in tumor markers or imaging, some individuals experiment with increasing their dose or combining their regimen with other supportive therapies, such as metabolic approaches or immune-boosting supplements.

It is also common for individuals to **cycle their use** of fenbendazole or ivermectin. Some protocols recommend **taking breaks** from treatment, such as using fenbendazole for three to six months, then pausing for a period before resuming. This is based on the theory that intermittent dosing may help prevent cancer cells from adapting to the treatment, though this remains an area of speculation rather than proven science.

Balancing Experimental Use with Conventional Monitoring

Because these medications are still being investigated for cancer treatment, regular medical monitoring is essential. Even individuals pursuing alternative or adjunctive approaches should continue working with their oncologists to track progress and make informed decisions. Bloodwork, imaging, and physical assessments can help ensure that the protocol is supporting overall health rather than causing unintended harm.

Ultimately, adjusting a fenbendazole or ivermectin protocol is a highly individualized process. While anecdotal success stories provide valuable insight, every person's cancer responds differently. The key to making these treatments as safe and effective as possible lies in careful observation, informed decision-making, and a willingness to adapt based on real-time results.

Chapter 5: Integrating the Protocol with Conventional and Alternative Therapies

Combining with Chemotherapy or Radiation

One of the biggest questions surrounding fenbendazole and ivermectin as potential cancer treatments is how they interact with conventional therapies like chemotherapy and radiation. Many individuals exploring these drugs are already undergoing traditional cancer treatments and want to know whether they can be safely combined. While formal clinical data is lacking, preliminary research and anecdotal reports suggest that these medications may **enhance** the effects of chemotherapy and radiation in certain cases rather than interfere with them.

Fenbendazole, for example, has been compared to certain chemotherapy drugs that **target microtubules**—the structural components that cancer cells rely on to divide. Some chemotherapy drugs, like paclitaxel and vinblastine, work by disrupting microtubules, preventing cancer cells from multiplying. Since fenbendazole appears to work through a similar mechanism, researchers have speculated that it might **increase the effectiveness of chemotherapy** when used alongside it.

Additionally, some laboratory studies suggest that fenbendazole may make cancer cells **more sensitive to radiation therapy**. Radiation kills cancer by damaging the DNA inside tumor cells, but some cancers develop resistance over time. Early research indicates that fenbendazole could weaken cancer cells' ability to repair themselves after radiation exposure, potentially increasing treatment effectiveness.

Ivermectin's Potential Role in Enhancing Standard Therapies

Ivermectin has also shown promise as a **chemosensitizer**, meaning it may help make cancer cells more responsive to chemotherapy drugs. Studies have suggested that ivermectin **interferes with drug resistance mechanisms**, particularly in cancers that have stopped responding to conventional treatment. Some cancers develop resistance by pumping chemotherapy drugs out of the cell before they can cause damage. Ivermectin has been found to **block these drug transporters**, effectively keeping chemotherapy inside cancer cells longer and increasing its impact.

There is also evidence that ivermectin can help **reduce inflammation and suppress cancer-supporting pathways**, which may enhance the effectiveness of both chemotherapy and immunotherapy. Some researchers believe that by **lowering inflammation and strengthening immune responses**, ivermectin may create a more hostile environment for cancer cells, making them easier to destroy with standard treatments.

Potential Risks and Considerations

While the potential benefits of combining fenbendazole or ivermectin with chemotherapy and radiation are intriguing, there are also important risks to consider. Since these drugs have not been extensively studied in this context, their interactions with specific chemotherapy agents are not well understood. Some questions that remain unanswered include:

- Could fenbendazole or ivermectin **increase side effects** when combined with chemotherapy?
- Do these drugs affect how the liver **metabolizes chemotherapy drugs**, potentially altering their effectiveness?
- Could ivermectin's impact on the immune system interfere with certain cancer treatments, such as immunotherapy?

Because of these unknowns, individuals considering combining these treatments should work closely with a healthcare professional who is open to discussing repurposed drugs. Regular **blood tests and imaging scans** can help track progress and catch any potential issues early.

For those already undergoing chemotherapy or radiation, a cautious approach may involve **starting with low doses** of fenbendazole or ivermectin and slowly increasing based on tolerance and response. By closely monitoring changes in symptoms, side effects, and tumor markers, individuals can make informed decisions about whether these drugs are a useful addition to their treatment plan.

While more research is needed to confirm the best way to combine fenbendazole and ivermectin with standard cancer treatments, the early findings suggest they may provide an additional layer of support, particularly for patients facing drug-resistant cancers or aggressive disease progression.

Potential Synergies with Natural Remedies

While fenbendazole and ivermectin are being explored as potential cancer treatments, many individuals incorporate natural therapies alongside these medications to further support their health. Alternative treatments such as **dietary strategies, herbal supplements, and metabolic therapies** are often used to create an environment in the body that makes it harder for cancer to thrive. Though scientific research on many of these approaches is still developing, there is growing evidence that certain natural remedies may work synergistically with repurposed drugs like fenbendazole and ivermectin.

One of the most widely studied complementary approaches is the **ketogenic diet**, which focuses on reducing carbohydrate intake and increasing healthy fats. Since many cancer cells rely heavily on glucose for fuel, lowering blood sugar levels through diet may help **starve tumors of their preferred energy source**. Some researchers believe that combining a ketogenic diet with metabolic-disrupting drugs like fenbendazole could enhance its effects, making cancer cells more vulnerable to treatment.

Another well-known natural therapy is **fasting or intermittent fasting**, which has been studied for its ability to put stress on cancer cells while protecting normal cells. Some individuals use fasting cycles to enhance the effectiveness of repurposed drugs, believing that a **fasted state may**

amplify the impact of treatments like ivermectin and fenbendazole by increasing autophagy—the body's process of breaking down damaged cells.

Herbs and Supplements That May Enhance Treatment

Several **herbal compounds and nutritional supplements** have been studied for their potential anti-cancer properties, and some may work in combination with fenbendazole and ivermectin.

- **Curcumin (from turmeric):** Well-known for its anti-inflammatory and anti-cancer properties, curcumin has been found to inhibit tumor growth and may enhance the effects of chemotherapy and repurposed drugs.
- **Berberine:** A plant-based compound that has shown potential in disrupting cancer metabolism, similar to how metformin works. Some individuals combine berberine with ivermectin to target energy pathways in cancer cells.

- **Quercetin:** A flavonoid that has demonstrated anti-tumor effects and may help suppress cancer cell signaling pathways.
- **Resveratrol:** Found in grapes and red wine, resveratrol has been studied for its ability to promote apoptosis (cell death) in cancer cells.
- **Green tea extract (EGCG):** A powerful antioxidant that has shown promise in reducing inflammation and supporting immune function in cancer patients.

While these supplements show promise, it is important to be aware of **potential interactions with conventional treatments**. Some natural compounds can interfere with chemotherapy drugs or enhance their toxicity, so individuals undergoing standard cancer treatment should consult with a knowledgeable practitioner before incorporating them into their regimen.

Building a Holistic Strategy

The key to integrating natural therapies with fenbendazole and ivermectin is to focus on

creating an internal environment that supports overall health while making it more difficult for cancer cells to survive. This includes:

- **Optimizing nutrition** to reduce inflammation and improve immune function.
- **Balancing metabolic pathways** through fasting or low-carb dietary approaches.
- **Incorporating anti-cancer supplements** that work alongside repurposed drugs.
- **Managing stress and sleep**, since chronic stress can weaken the immune system and promote tumor growth.

While alternative approaches should never replace evidence-based medical treatments, they may serve as powerful **adjunct therapies** that support the body's ability to fight cancer. As research into repurposed drugs and metabolic strategies continues, the hope is that these integrated approaches will become more widely studied and accepted as part of a comprehensive cancer treatment plan.

Addressing Drug Interactions

While fenbendazole and ivermectin are being explored for their potential role in cancer treatment, understanding their interactions with other medications is crucial for ensuring safety and effectiveness. Many individuals using these drugs are also undergoing conventional treatments such as chemotherapy, radiation, or immunotherapy, all of which involve complex metabolic pathways. Taking multiple treatments simultaneously can sometimes lead to unintended effects, either by **reducing the effectiveness of certain drugs or increasing the risk of side effects**.

One of the key concerns with drug interactions is how these medications are **processed by the liver**. The liver is responsible for metabolizing most drugs, and some medications can either speed up or slow down this process, leading to altered drug levels in the body.

Fenbendazole and Drug Metabolism

Fenbendazole is primarily broken down by the liver, specifically through **cytochrome P450 enzymes**, which are responsible for processing many pharmaceutical drugs. This means that certain medications that also rely on these enzymes—such as some chemotherapy agents, blood thinners, or immunosuppressants—could potentially be affected when taken alongside fenbendazole.

Medications that may interact with fenbendazole include:

- **Certain chemotherapy drugs** – Some reports suggest that fenbendazole may enhance the effects of microtubule-targeting chemotherapy drugs like paclitaxel and vinblastine, but more research is needed.
- **Blood thinners (anticoagulants)** – Since fenbendazole is processed through liver enzymes, there is a possibility it could alter the effectiveness of medications like warfarin.
- **Immunosuppressants** – Drugs used in organ transplants or autoimmune

conditions may have altered metabolism when combined with fenbendazole. While no major adverse interactions have been widely reported, individuals taking fenbendazole alongside prescription medications should **consult with a healthcare professional and monitor for any unexpected side effects**.

Ivermectin and Potential Interactions

Ivermectin also undergoes liver metabolism, specifically through **CYP3A4**, an enzyme responsible for breaking down many drugs. This means that any medication that affects CYP3A4 levels—either increasing or decreasing its activity—could impact how ivermectin is processed in the body.

Drugs that may interact with ivermectin include:

- **Certain antibiotics (e.g., erythromycin, clarithromycin)** – These can slow ivermectin metabolism, increasing its concentration in the bloodstream and

potentially leading to neurological side effects.
- **Anti-seizure medications (e.g., carbamazepine, phenytoin)** – These drugs can speed up the breakdown of ivermectin, potentially reducing its effectiveness.
- **HIV and antiviral medications** – Some protease inhibitors used for HIV treatment may alter ivermectin metabolism.
- **Immunotherapy drugs** – Since ivermectin has some immune-modulating properties, there is speculation that it could either enhance or interfere with certain immunotherapies, though more research is needed.

Another factor to consider is **neurological sensitivity**. In rare cases, individuals with a genetic mutation affecting the **P-glycoprotein (P-gp) transporter** may experience heightened neurological effects when taking ivermectin. This is because P-gp helps regulate drug entry into the brain, and when it is not functioning properly, ivermectin levels can build up, potentially causing dizziness, confusion, or other side effects.

Minimizing Risks and Monitoring for Reactions

Since there is limited formal research on how fenbendazole and ivermectin interact with other cancer treatments, the best approach is to **start with conservative dosing, closely monitor symptoms, and communicate with a healthcare provider**. Individuals using these drugs should:

- **Track symptoms** – Noticing changes such as increased fatigue, dizziness, or unexpected side effects may indicate a drug interaction.
- **Space out medications** – Some individuals take fenbendazole or ivermectin at different times of day than their prescription drugs to minimize metabolic interference.
- **Check liver function** – Since both drugs are processed through the liver, periodic blood tests may help ensure that liver enzymes remain stable.

While the potential for drug interactions exists, many individuals successfully integrate fenbendazole and ivermectin into their treatment plans with careful management. As more research emerges, a clearer understanding of how these drugs interact with conventional treatments will help refine their role in cancer care.

Long-Term Use vs. Short-Term Protocols

One of the biggest questions surrounding fenbendazole and ivermectin in cancer treatment is whether they should be used **continuously** or in **cycles**. Since these medications were not originally designed for cancer, no formal guidelines exist on how long they should be taken or whether breaks are necessary. Individuals using these drugs off-label often rely on anecdotal experiences, adjusting their protocols based on how their bodies respond.

The Case for Long-Term Use

Some individuals choose to take fenbendazole or ivermectin continuously, believing that stopping might allow cancer cells to regain their strength. The rationale behind this approach is that cancer often adapts to treatments, and maintaining steady pressure on tumors may help prevent resistance from developing.

For example, fenbendazole disrupts microtubule function in cancer cells, much like certain chemotherapy drugs. Since chemotherapy is often administered over extended periods, some believe that a **consistent intake of fenbendazole** may produce a similar anti-cancer effect.

Ivermectin, on the other hand, has been studied for its ability to regulate metabolic pathways and immune responses. Some researchers speculate that its **immune-modulating effects** may take time to build, making continuous use beneficial for those trying to maintain a long-term defense against cancer.

The Case for Cycling Protocols

Others prefer to **cycle their use** of fenbendazole and ivermectin, meaning they take the drugs for a set period, then pause before resuming. This approach is based on the theory that intermittent dosing may help prevent toxicity, allow the body to reset, and even enhance effectiveness by keeping cancer cells from adapting.

Common cycling strategies include:

- **Fenbendazole "3 days on, 4 days off"** – This was the original protocol followed by Joe Tippens, and many continue to use it.
- **Ivermectin 5 days on, 2 days off** – Some individuals follow this schedule, while others use it for a few weeks and then take a break.
- **Alternating months** – Some people take fenbendazole or ivermectin for 30 days, then stop for a few weeks before resuming.

The idea behind cycling is that tumors may become resistant to continuous exposure, much like bacteria develop resistance to antibiotics. By giving the body short breaks, proponents of this method believe it may keep cancer cells from adapting to the treatment.

How to Decide?

Since there is no definitive answer, the decision between **continuous vs. cyclical use** depends on several factors:

- **Response to treatment** – Individuals who see positive effects (such as tumor shrinkage or stable scans) may choose to continue uninterrupted.
- **Side effects** – If someone experiences fatigue, brain fog, or digestive issues, cycling may allow the body time to recover.
- **Cancer type and stage** – Some aggressive cancers may require continuous suppression, while slow-growing tumors may not need constant treatment.

Many individuals adjust their protocols over time, based on **tumor marker tests, imaging results, and overall well-being**. Those with **stable disease** may eventually reduce their dosage or transition to a **maintenance protocol**, taking the drugs at a lower frequency to prevent recurrence.

While long-term safety data is lacking, many people have successfully incorporated fenbendazole and ivermectin into their cancer-fighting regimens for months or even years without major issues. The key is **consistent monitoring and adjusting the approach as needed** to balance effectiveness with overall health.

Personalized Treatment Plans

Every cancer case is unique, and what works for one person may not be the best approach for another. Factors like cancer type, stage, genetic profile, overall health, and current treatments all influence how a patient responds to different therapies. Because fenbendazole and ivermectin are being used off-label, individuals who incorporate them into their treatment strategy often develop **personalized protocols** based on their specific needs, symptoms, and response to treatment.

Tailoring the Protocol to Cancer Type and Stage

One of the biggest factors influencing a treatment plan is **cancer aggressiveness**. Fast-growing cancers, such as certain **lung, pancreatic, and brain cancers**, often require **continuous treatment with higher doses**, whereas slower-growing cancers may allow for a more cyclical approach.

- **Aggressive cancers** – Individuals facing advanced or fast-growing cancers may choose to take fenbendazole and ivermectin **daily** with minimal breaks, aiming to maintain constant pressure on tumor growth.
- **Slow-growing cancers** – For cancers that progress more gradually, some individuals experiment with **cycling protocols** (such as alternating weeks or taking periodic breaks) to balance effectiveness with overall health.

For those undergoing **conventional treatments**, the timing of fenbendazole or ivermectin use may also vary. Some people choose to take these drugs **during chemotherapy or radiation** to enhance their effects, while others wait until conventional treatment is completed before adding them to their routine.

Adjusting Based on Health and Tolerance

Not everyone responds to treatment in the same way. Some individuals tolerate fenbendazole and ivermectin with no noticeable side effects, while others may experience fatigue, digestive discomfort, or neurological symptoms like dizziness.

- **For those with strong tolerance:** Continuous use or higher doses may be an option.
- **For those experiencing side effects:** Lower doses or intermittent schedules (e.g., five days on, two days off) may be a better fit.

Other health conditions also play a role. People with **liver or kidney disease** should be cautious, as these drugs are metabolized through the liver. Regular blood tests can help ensure that **liver enzymes remain stable** and that no organ stress is occurring.

Tracking Progress and Making Adjustments

Since there is no universal dosing guideline for using fenbendazole or ivermectin in cancer, individuals must often rely on their own **monitoring and tracking** to assess effectiveness. Some ways to measure progress include:

- **Tumor marker blood tests** – Checking levels like CA-125 (ovarian cancer), PSA (prostate cancer), or CEA (colon cancer) can indicate whether treatment is making an impact.
- **Imaging scans** – MRIs, CT scans, or PET scans at regular intervals can reveal changes in tumor size or spread.
- **Physical symptoms** – Some individuals report decreased pain, improved energy, or overall well-being after using these drugs, though this varies.

If a treatment appears to be working, some individuals continue their regimen unchanged. If there is **no noticeable improvement**, adjustments may be made—such as increasing the dosage, adding synergistic supplements, or exploring other metabolic approaches like fasting or dietary changes.

The most effective cancer treatment plans are highly individualized. By combining **scientific research, personal tracking, and professional guidance**, individuals can create a plan that best fits their needs, balancing safety with the potential for improved outcomes.

Chapter 6: The Future of Repurposed Drugs in Cancer Treatment

The Rise of Drug Repurposing

The search for effective cancer treatments has traditionally focused on developing new drugs, often at great expense and over long periods of time. However, an increasing number of scientists and medical professionals are turning to an alternative approach: **drug repurposing**—the process of identifying new therapeutic uses for existing medications. This strategy has gained attention not only because it saves time and money but also because it can bring potentially life-saving treatments to patients much faster.

Many of today's most well-known drugs were originally intended for completely different conditions. For example:

- **Metformin**, the common diabetes drug, is now being studied for its anti-cancer properties.

- **Aspirin**, originally used for pain relief, is widely recommended for heart disease prevention and has also been linked to reduced cancer risk.
- **Thalidomide**, once infamous for causing birth defects, was later found to be an effective treatment for multiple myeloma.

Fenbendazole and ivermectin fit into this same category—drugs with well-documented safety profiles that were initially designed for other purposes but may have unexpected cancer-fighting abilities. If these medications prove to be effective, they could represent **low-cost, widely available options** for patients who need alternatives to conventional treatments.

Why Some Drugs Get Overlooked

Despite the potential benefits of repurposing existing drugs, many promising treatments struggle to gain mainstream acceptance. The primary reason is **lack of financial incentive**. Pharmaceutical companies invest billions of dollars into drug development, and they recoup these costs through patents that give them exclusive rights to sell a new medication for a set period.

Once a drug like fenbendazole or ivermectin is off-patent, it becomes **cheap and widely accessible**, meaning there is little profit to be made from funding large-scale clinical trials. This creates a significant barrier to getting repurposed drugs formally approved for new indications, even when preliminary research is promising.

Additionally, **medical institutions tend to favor established protocols**. Oncologists are trained to follow standard treatment guidelines, which are based on **clinical trial data and regulatory approvals**. Because fenbendazole and ivermectin have not undergone large-scale human trials for cancer, many doctors are reluctant to recommend them, even when patients express interest.

The Growing Movement for Alternative Cancer Treatments

Despite these challenges, a growing number of patients, independent researchers, and integrative practitioners are advocating for the exploration of repurposed drugs in cancer treatment. Online communities and patient support groups have played a significant role in spreading awareness, sharing success stories, and pushing for further research.

While mainstream medicine is often slow to adopt new approaches, history has shown that **patient-driven demand** can help accelerate change. If enough individuals report positive outcomes and scientific research continues to build, repurposed drugs like fenbendazole and ivermectin may eventually be recognized as legitimate treatment options.

The next step in this process is expanding the evidence base through **well-structured clinical trials** and ensuring that patients have access to **unbiased information** so they can make informed decisions about their care. As drug repurposing continues to gain traction, the hope is that more affordable and accessible treatment options will become available for those who need them most.

The Challenge of Gaining Medical Acceptance

Despite the growing interest in repurposed drugs like fenbendazole and ivermectin, getting them formally recognized as cancer treatments remains a major challenge. The process of integrating new therapies into standard oncology protocols is slow, heavily regulated, and often influenced by financial and institutional factors.

One of the biggest obstacles is the **lack of large-scale clinical trials**. For a drug to be officially approved for cancer treatment, it must go through a rigorous testing process that includes:

- **Preclinical research** (lab and animal studies) to establish basic mechanisms.
- **Phase 1 trials** to test safety in humans.
- **Phase 2 trials** to assess effectiveness in small patient groups.

- **Phase 3 trials** involving large numbers of patients to confirm benefits and compare against existing treatments.

Since fenbendazole and ivermectin are already off-patent, pharmaceutical companies have little incentive to fund these expensive trials. Without industry backing, the responsibility for research often falls to **independent scientists, universities, and non-profit organizations**, which have fewer resources and face greater difficulties in launching large studies.

Resistance from the Medical Community

Most oncologists follow **standard treatment guidelines**, which are based on clinical trial data, regulatory approvals, and recommendations from institutions like the FDA, the National Cancer Institute (NCI), and the American Society of Clinical Oncology (ASCO). Because fenbendazole and ivermectin have not been formally studied in large human cancer trials, they are not included in these guidelines, making many doctors hesitant to recommend them.

Some medical professionals are also wary of **patient-led experimentation**, believing that off-label use of repurposed drugs carries risks. Since dosing, drug interactions, and long-term effects have not been well-studied in the context of cancer, doctors worry that unsupervised use could lead to unforeseen complications. However, this caution can sometimes translate into **dismissal or unwillingness to discuss alternative options**, leaving patients to seek out treatments on their own.

Pushing for Greater Acceptance

For repurposed drugs to gain medical recognition, several things need to happen:

- **More published research** – Small studies and case reports have begun appearing in scientific journals, but larger-scale trials are needed to validate findings.
- **Physician awareness and education** – Some oncologists are open to repurposed drugs but lack knowledge about their potential benefits. Increased medical

education on drug repurposing could help bridge this gap.
- **Patient advocacy** – Many advances in cancer treatment have been driven by **patient demand**. The more individuals push for research and transparency, the harder it becomes to ignore potential therapies.
- **Regulatory flexibility** – Some countries are beginning to recognize the value of repurposed drugs and may develop **faster approval pathways** for medications with strong safety profiles.

While mainstream medicine is often slow to change, history has shown that new treatments—especially those driven by patient interest—can eventually break through resistance. The key is persistence, continued research, and a commitment to making effective, affordable treatments accessible to all.

Advocacy and the Role of Independent Researchers

While large pharmaceutical companies often drive medical advancements, many promising treatments emerge from **independent researchers, patient communities, and small-scale studies**. The exploration of fenbendazole and ivermectin as potential cancer treatments has largely been fueled by grassroots efforts rather than industry-backed research. As a result, **advocacy and independent inquiry have become essential in pushing these treatments toward greater medical recognition**.

In recent years, patient-driven initiatives have become more influential in shaping research priorities. Platforms such as **Crowdfunded Science and Independent Research Networks** have allowed scientists to pursue studies that might not receive traditional funding. These efforts have helped launch trials on drug repurposing, including investigations into older medications that may have been overlooked due to financial disincentives.

Patient advocacy groups have also played a significant role in **pressuring regulatory agencies** to consider alternative treatments. Historically, movements led by patients have helped accelerate research and approval for new therapies. For example:

- **The HIV/AIDS community in the 1980s** successfully pushed for faster drug approvals and wider access to experimental treatments.
- **Parents of children with rare diseases** have driven the creation of expanded drug access programs.
- **Cancer patient networks** have organized to fund independent research on alternative and repurposed therapies.

A similar pattern is emerging with fenbendazole and ivermectin. As more patients report benefits, their stories create momentum that encourages researchers to investigate further. Some oncologists and integrative medicine practitioners are now beginning to acknowledge the potential of repurposed drugs, though acceptance remains limited within mainstream medicine.

Bridging the Gap Between Alternative and Conventional Medicine

One of the challenges in promoting repurposed drugs is overcoming the **divide between conventional oncology and alternative medicine**. Many patients who seek out fenbendazole or ivermectin do so after exhausting traditional treatments, often turning to online communities for guidance. However, without medical oversight, **patients may struggle to navigate proper dosing, safety considerations, and potential interactions with other treatments**.

Bridging this gap requires collaboration between **forward-thinking medical professionals and patient-led research efforts**. Some doctors specializing in integrative oncology have begun incorporating repurposed drugs into their protocols, combining them with metabolic therapies, diet modifications, and immune-supporting supplements. This approach allows patients to use experimental treatments **while remaining under medical**

supervision, ensuring better tracking of progress and safety.

Ultimately, the future of repurposed drug research depends on **continued advocacy, independent research, and increased awareness within the medical community**. While acceptance may be slow, the persistence of researchers, doctors, and patients alike is creating a shift in how alternative treatments are viewed. If more studies confirm the potential of fenbendazole and ivermectin, these medications could one day become recognized as **legitimate, low-cost options** for cancer treatment.

Ongoing and Future Trials to Watch

As interest in drug repurposing grows, researchers are beginning to investigate fenbendazole and ivermectin more seriously in clinical settings. While much of the current evidence is based on laboratory studies and anecdotal reports, several ongoing and planned trials may soon provide **more**

definitive answers about their potential role in cancer treatment.

One of the most promising areas of research involves **ivermectin's effect on drug-resistant cancers**. Some studies suggest that ivermectin may help overcome **chemotherapy resistance**, particularly in aggressive cancers like triple-negative breast cancer and pancreatic cancer. A recent trial at the **University of Texas MD Anderson Cancer Center** is evaluating ivermectin's ability to enhance the effects of standard chemotherapy drugs by blocking survival pathways that cancer cells rely on. If successful, this study could pave the way for larger clinical trials.

Fenbendazole, on the other hand, has not yet been the subject of major human trials, but **researchers in Europe and Asia** have begun exploring its potential through smaller pilot studies. Some of these focus on its ability to **disrupt cancer metabolism** and act as a microtubule inhibitor, similar to established chemotherapy agents. A team at **the National**

Cancer Institute (NCI) has reportedly expressed interest in further studying fenbendazole, though no large-scale trials have been confirmed.

What These Trials Aim to Prove

For fenbendazole and ivermectin to gain mainstream acceptance, researchers will need to demonstrate several key factors:

- **Efficacy** – Do these drugs significantly slow tumor growth, shrink tumors, or improve survival rates in human patients?
- **Optimal Dosage** – What dose is needed to achieve anti-cancer effects without causing side effects?
- **Safety in Cancer Patients** – Since these drugs were not originally designed for cancer, trials must confirm that they are safe for long-term use in this context.
- **Potential Synergies** – Do fenbendazole and ivermectin work best on their own, or in combination with existing cancer therapies like chemotherapy, radiation, or immunotherapy?

One of the biggest hurdles is securing **funding for these trials**, as most pharmaceutical companies are reluctant to invest in studying non-patentable drugs. Instead, much of the research is being driven by **universities, independent researchers, and patient advocacy groups** who are pushing for more investigation into these low-cost alternatives.

How Patients Can Stay Informed

For those interested in following the latest research, several resources track drug repurposing studies and ongoing clinical trials:

- **ClinicalTrials.gov** – A database of registered clinical trials worldwide, where new studies on fenbendazole and ivermectin may be posted.
- **The Repurposing Drugs in Oncology (ReDO) Project** – A research initiative focused on investigating existing drugs for cancer treatment.
- **Patient advocacy groups** – Online communities and forums often share

updates on emerging research and real-world patient experiences.

While the research on fenbendazole and ivermectin is still in its early stages, the growing number of studies suggests that **more concrete data may be available in the coming years**. If ongoing trials confirm their effectiveness, these drugs could eventually become **widely accepted and integrated into cancer treatment protocols**, offering patients a **low-cost, accessible alternative** to traditional therapies.

Final Thoughts and Encouragement

The search for effective cancer treatments is constantly evolving, and repurposed drugs like fenbendazole and ivermectin represent a new frontier in oncology—one that challenges the traditional pharmaceutical model and gives hope to patients seeking alternative options. While these medications were never originally intended to treat cancer, the growing body of anecdotal evidence, laboratory research, and emerging clinical studies suggests that they may hold **real potential** in helping to slow tumor growth, improve treatment outcomes, and even enhance conventional therapies.

For those navigating a cancer diagnosis, the sheer volume of information—both scientific and anecdotal—can be overwhelming. The key to making informed decisions is to **approach new treatments with an open but cautious mindset**. While many have reported success using fenbendazole and ivermectin, it is important to recognize that cancer is a complex disease with many variables. What works for one person may not work for another, and **tracking progress, consulting knowledgeable healthcare professionals, and staying informed on emerging research** are essential steps for those considering these therapies.

The world of drug repurposing is still in its early stages, but the increasing interest in fenbendazole, ivermectin, and other overlooked medications is a sign that change may be on the horizon. As more **scientists,**

independent researchers, and patient advocates push for further study, these treatments may eventually gain broader medical acceptance, leading to **wider accessibility and formal guidelines for safe and effective use**.

For now, the most important takeaway is that **hope exists in many forms**. Whether through conventional treatments, alternative approaches, or a combination of both, the pursuit of better cancer care is ongoing. Those who explore repurposed drugs should do so with careful research, proper monitoring, and a willingness to adjust their approach based on new evidence.

The future of cancer treatment may not come solely from expensive new drugs, but from **re-examining the medicines we already have**—and that possibility is one worth fighting for.

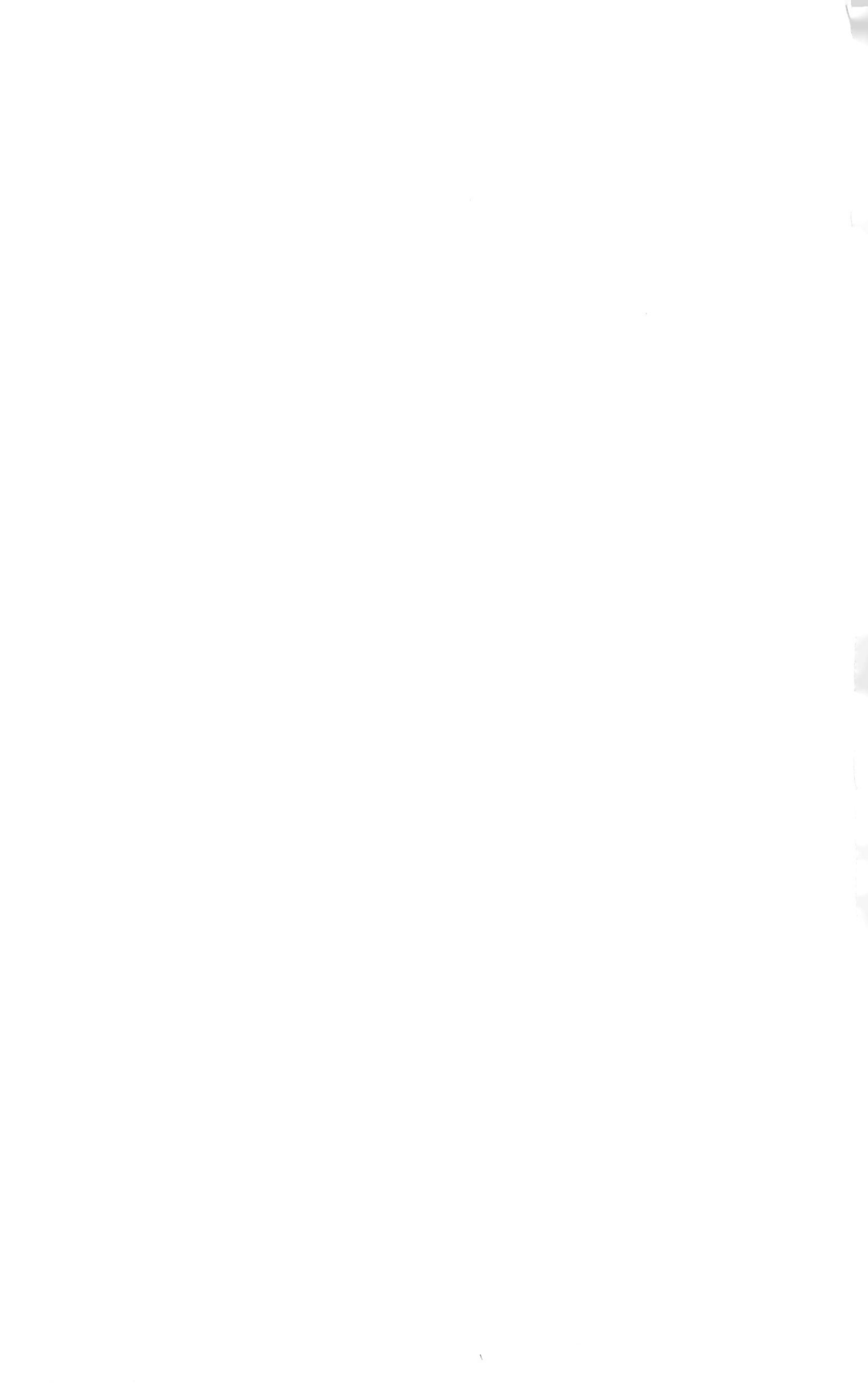

Made in United States
Troutdale, OR
05/26/2025